GARY W STIDHAM

CPR / AED

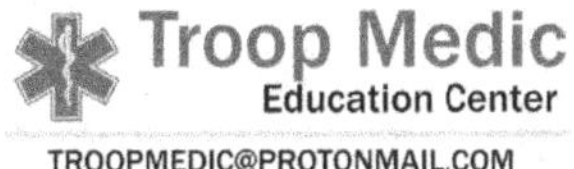

Troop Medic
Education Center
TROOPMEDIC@PROTONMAIL.COM

Contents

First Aid

The primary goal of first aid is to prevent death or serious injury from worsening.

Preserve life - The overriding aim of all medical care, which includes first aid, is to save lives and minimize the threat of death. First aid done correctly should help reduce the patient's level of pain and calm them down during the evaluation and treatment process.

Prevent further harm - Prevention of further harm includes addressing both external factors, such as moving a patient away from any cause of harm, and applying first aid techniques to prevent worsening of the condition, such as applying pressure to stop a bleed.

Promote recovery - First aid also involves trying to start the recovery process from the illness or injury. The first thing that anyone providing first aid should be aware of when entering a situation is the potential for danger to themselves. This is especially important in first aid, as situations which have been dangerous to others carry an inherent risk of danger to those providing first aid.

Environmental danger - A danger in the surroundings, such as falling objects, broken glass/debris, fast vehicles, chemicals, animals, etc.

Human danger - Danger from people at the scene (including the victim) which can be intentional or accidental. Keeping yourself protected is the first priority of any first responder.

The key is to always be aware of your surroundings and the situation, and be alert for any changes therein. Once you are aware of the hazards, you can then take steps to minimize the risk to oneself. One of the key dangers to a first responder is bodily fluids, such as blood, vomit, urine and feces, all of which pose a risk of cross contamination. Body fluids and feces can carry infections and diseases. The main tool of the first responder to avoid this risk is a pair of impermeable gloves. Gloves protect the key contact point with the victim and allow you to work safety. They protect from bodily fluids and feces, or parasites that the victim may have. The other key piece of protective equipment that should be in every first aid kit is an adjunct for helping to perform safe mouth-to-mouth resuscitation.

Good Samaritan Laws

Good Samaritan laws in the United States and Canada are laws that reduce the liability to those who choose to aid others who are injured or ill. Though it does not protect you from being sued, it just significantly reduces your liability. They are intended to reduce bystanders' hesitation to assist for fear of being prosecuted for unintentional injury or wrongful death. Typically, the Good Samaritan legislation does not cover an individual who exceeds their training level or scope of practice; nor would you be protected against gross negligence. At minimum, call the local emergency number.

General Guidelines

Unless a caretaker relationship (such as a parent-child or doctor-patient relationship) exists prior to the illness or injury, or the "Good Samaritan" is responsible for the existence of the illness or injury, no person is required to give aid of any sort to a victim. Any first aid provided must not be in exchange for any reward or financial compensation. As a result, medical professionals are typically not protected by Good Samaritan laws when performing first aid in connection with their employment.

If aid begins, the responder must not leave the scene until:

- It is necessary in order to call for needed medical assistance.
- Somebody of equal or higher ability can take over.

- Continuing to give aid is unsafe (this can be as simple as a lack of adequate protection against potential diseases, such as vinyl, latex or nitrile gloves to protect against blood-borne pathogens) as a responder can never be forced to put himself or herself in danger to aid another person.

The responder is not legally liable for the death, disfigurement or disability of the victim as long as the responder acted rationally, in good faith, and in accordance with their level of training.

Assisting with medications can be a vital component during a medical emergency. Assisting, does not imply actually administering the medication—this is an advanced level skill, which, if done, may open you up to liability from going beyond your level of training.

PROFESSIONAL RESCUERS (Healthcare Providers, Medical staff, Lifeguards, etc.) have what is known as a duty to act and are bound to provide help. Individuals with a duty to act need the knowledge and skills to respond appropriately to breathing and cardiac emergencies until more advanced medical personnel arrive and take over. This includes CPR and the use of an automated external defibrillator (AED) to care for a person experiencing cardiac arrest.

Consent

The simplest way to gain consent is to ask the victim if they will allow you to treat them. Talk to the victim and build up a rapport with them. During this conversation, it is important to identify the following key points:

- **Who you are** - start with your name and explain that you are a trained first responder.
- **Why you are with them** - they likely know they have an injury or illness, (although you can't always assume this in the case of patients in emotional shock, children or those with learning difficulties) but explain to them that you would like to help with their injury or illness.
- **What you are going to do** - some first aid procedures can be uncomfortable (such as the sting which accompanies cleaning a wound with saline), so it is important to be honest with the patient about what you are doing, and if necessary, why it is important.

There are some cases where you can assume that the victim gives their consent to you treating them. The key reason for assuming consent is if the patient is unconscious or has a very reduced level of consciousness. In these cases, you can perform any reasonable treatment within your level of training, and your position is protected in most jurisdictions.

There are also some cases where the first responder may have to exercise a level of judgment in treating a victim who may initially refuse. Cases like this include when the victim is:

- Intoxicated or irrational (i.e. delusional, insane or confused due to the injuries)
- A minor (parent or guardian must give consent if present and able)
- Suffering from learning difficulties. In these judgment cases, the first responder must make a decision, even if the victim is refusing treatment. If this occurs, it is very important to make a note of the decision, why it was taken, and why it was believed that the person was unfit to refuse treatment.

It is advisable to summon professional medical assistance if you believe the victim should be treated and is refusing, as medical professionals are experienced in dealing with people reluctant to accept treatment.

In some cases, relatives may object to the treatment of their relative. In the first instance, it may not be any decision of the relative to choose to consent to first aid treatment. In most countries, the only time this decision can be definitively taken is if the person requiring treatment is a child. The other main consideration is if the person claiming to refuse consent on behalf of the victim is in fact a relative, or if they have the victim's best interests at heart. In some cases, the person may have caused harm to the victim. If in this case, and you fear for your safety, or the person becomes aggressive, you should look after your own safety as a priority and call for assistance from the police.

In other cases, the presumption for the first responder must be towards treating the victim, especially if they are unconscious.

Some victims may have a statement recorded, called an advanced directive or living will, that they do not wish to be treated in the case of life threatening illness.

The first responder should always presume towards treating a victim, allowing health care professionals to make the final decision. Almost every first aid treatment will only extend life, rather than definitively save it, meaning you are usually not breaking the advance directive.

Heart Attack

Heart Attack Symptoms

Though not all of the warning signs occur in every attack and can vary based on your gender and age, and if you have diabetes, a person should seek medical attention right away if any of these symptoms occur:

- Uncomfortable pressure, fullness, squeezing, or pain in the center of the chest that lasts more than a few minutes or goes away and comes back
- Pain spreading to the shoulders, neck, back, jaw, and arms
- Chest discomfort with lightheadedness, fainting, sweating, or nausea
- Shortness of breath with or without chest discomfort
- Feeling very anxious or very tired
- Breaking out in a cold sweat

Men and women may have different symptoms, but chest pressure or pain is still the most common heart attack symptom for both genders. Women are somewhat more likely than men to have some of the other common symptoms, particularly shortness of breath, nausea/vomiting, and back or jaw pain. Older people may faint, which can be a sign of a heart attack. People with diabetes may not have chest pain at all.

If you suspect someone is having a heart attack:

- **Call 911** or your local number for emergencies. Tell the person who answers where you are and that someone is having a heart attack. Don't hang up until you're told to do so.
- Don't let someone who is having symptoms drive themselves to the hospital. If you are having symptoms, don't drive yourself.
- Be prepared to administer cardiopulmonary resuscitation (CPR), if necessary.
- If an automated external defibrillator (AED) is available, have it brought to the patient and make sure it is ready for use if needed.

Your primary role is to provide emotional support and arrange for prompt transport to an appropriate medical facility. Because the patient's emotional state can affect his or her physical condition, emotional support is valuable as it can help prevent cardiac arrest.

Giving one adult aspirin (325 mg) or 4 low-dose aspirins (81 mg each) may help to reduce the chance of death from a heart attack. Instruct the patient to chew the aspirin and then swallow it. However, be sure the patient is not allergic to aspirin and has not had any recent internal bleeding such as a stomach ulcer.

Heart Attack (myocardial infarction) results when one or more of the coronary arteries is completely blocked. The two primary causes of coronary artery blockage are severe atherosclerosis and a blood clot from somewhere else in the circulatory system that breaks free and lodges in the artery. If one of the coronary arteries becomes blocked, the part of the heart muscle served by that artery is deprived of oxygen and dies.

Blockage of a coronary artery causes the patient to experience immediate and severe pain. The pain of angina pectoris and a heart attack may be similar at first. Most heart attack patients describe the pain as crushing and the pain may
radiate from the chest to the left arm, to the jaw, or to the back.

Heart conditions do not cause all chest pain. It is better for the patient to treat the

pain as if it is a heart attack than to under treat the symptoms. The patient is

usually short of breath, weak, sweating, nauseated, and may vomit.

Nitroglycerin pills or spray will not relieve the pain of a heart attack. The pain

will persist, unlike the pain of angina, which rarely lasts more than 5 minutes.

Angina Pectoris

As atherosclerosis progresses in the coronary arteries, it can reduce the blood (oxygen) supply to the heart enough to cause pain or pressure in the chest. This pain is known as angina pectoris or simply angina; the heart needs more oxygen than the narrowed coronary arteries can deliver. When a patient has chest pain, first ask the person to describe the pain. Patients often describe angina as pressure or heavy discomfort. The patient may say something like, "It feels like an elephant is sitting on my chest." Angina attacks are usually brought on by exertion, emotion or eating. The patient may feel crushing pain in the chest. The pain may radiate to either or both arms, the neck, jaw or any combination of these sites. The patient is often short of breath and sweating, extremely frightened, and has a sense of doom. The patient may experience nausea and vomiting. Ask whether the patient is already being treated for a diagnosed heart condition; if the answer is "yes," ask if the patient has a pill or spray to take for angina pain. A patient who has experienced previous episodes of angina usually has medication that he or she can place or spray under the tongue to relieve the pain. The most common medication of this type is nitroglycerin.

Difference Between a Panic Attack and a Heart Attack

Location and Characterization of Pain

- With a heart attack, pain is classically felt below the breastbone as a dull pressure. It may radiate up to the neck and jaw or down the left arm. It is a vague pain you cannot specifically locate with the tip of your finger. Sharp pain or pain that you can point to with a finger is unlikely to be from the heart.
- Panic attacks, on the other hand, may cause chest pain with a sharp or stabbing sensation, or a choking sensation in the throat.

Never Ignore Chest Pain

Never ignore chest discomfort or assume it is from a panic attack, particularly if you have never been diagnosed with panic attacks.

Heartburn or Heart Attack

The symptoms of heartburn may mimic those of angina or a heart attack (or vice versa). If you're uncertain, don't hesitate to get to an emergency room for an evaluation as soon as possible.

COMMON SYMPTOMS

Angina or Heart Attack

- Tightness, pressure, squeezing, stabbing, or dull pain, most often in the center of the chest
- Pain that spreads to the shoulders, neck, or arms
- Irregular or rapid heartbeat
- Cold sweat or clammy skin
- Lightheadedness, weakness, or dizziness

- Shortness of breath
- Nausea, indigestion, and sometimes vomiting
- The appearance of symptoms with physical exertion or extreme stress

Heartburn / Gastroesophageal Reflux Disease (GERD)

- Burning chest pain that begins at the breastbone
- Pain that moves up toward your throat but doesn't typically radiate to your shoulders, neck, or arms
- Sensation that food is coming back into your mouth
- Bitter or acidic taste at the back of your throat
- Pain that worsens when you lie down or bend over
- The appearance of symptoms after a large or spicy meal

When in doubt, check it out

If you're not sure if it's heartburn or your heart, seek medical attention right away. It's very easy to confuse the two issues so let a doctor rule out the most severe possibility.

Stroke

- Stroke is the fifth leading cause of death in the U.S. and the leading cause of severe long-term disability. Someone dies of a stroke every four minutes in the U.S.
- 80% of all strokes result from a blockage or blood clot in a blood vessel in the brain.
- 20% of all strokes occur when an artery suddenly bursts and bleeds into or around the brain.
- Immediate treatment can limit or prevent brain damage from a stroke.

What is a Stroke

A stroke happens when something disrupts blood flow to an area of the brain. The extent of stroke damage depends on how much brain tissue is affected and how quickly the stroke is treated. Strokes can cause long-lasting disability or even death.

The most common type of stroke, an ischemic stroke, occurs when a blockage clogs an artery, starving the brain of oxygen and vital nutrients. A hemorrhagic stroke happens when an artery ruptures and blood spills into the brain.

When blood flow to the brain is suddenly disrupted, oxygen-starved tissue rapidly begins to die. Sudden confusion, visual disturbances, dizziness, an unusual headache, numbness, or weakness—especially on one side of the body—can signal the onset of a stroke.

Ischemic Stroke

An ischemic stroke is the most common stroke. A blood clot blocks an artery, starving the brain of oxygen and vital nutrients. Often the clogged artery is already narrowed by fatty deposits. A blood clot can also travel to the brain from another part of the body. If the blood supply is interrupted for more than a few minutes, the brain can suffer lasting injury.

Hemorrhagic (bleeding) Strokes

- **Intracerebral hemorrhage** is bleeding within the brain from a broken blood vessel. The immediate damaging effects of bleeding in the brain range from movement and speech problems to paralysis.
- **Subarachnoid hemorrhage** occurs when blood from a damaged blood vessel accumulates at the surface of the brain. When this happens, blood spills into the space between the brain and the skull.

People are at risk for pneumonia, blood clots, and other severe complications for several weeks after a bleeding stroke.

Symptoms of Stroke

Warning signs of a stroke

- **Trouble speaking and understanding what others are saying.** You may experience confusion, slur words or have difficulty understanding speech.
- **Paralysis or numbness of the face, arm or leg.** You may develop sudden numbness, weakness or paralysis in the face, arm or leg; this often affects just one side of the body. Try to raise both your arms over your head at the same time; if one arm begins to fall, you may be having a stroke. Also,

one side of your mouth may droop when you try to smile.

- **Problems seeing in one or both eyes.** You may suddenly have blurred or blackened vision in one or both eyes, or you may see double.
- **Headache.** A sudden, severe headache, which may be accompanied by vomiting, dizziness or altered consciousness, may indicate that you're having a stroke.
- **Trouble walking.** You may stumble or lose your balance. You may also have sudden dizziness or a loss of coordination.

Seek immediate medical attention if you notice any signs or symptoms of a stroke, even if they seem to come and go or they disappear completely. Think **"FAST"** and do the following:

- **Face.** Ask the person to smile. Does one side of the face droop?
- **Arms.** Ask the person to raise both arms. Does one arm drift downward? Or is one arm unable to rise?
- **Speech.** Ask the person to repeat a simple phrase. Is his or her speech slurred or strange?
- **Time.** If you observe any of these signs, call 911 or emergency medical help immediately.

Call 911 right away! Don't wait to see if symptoms stop- every minute counts. The longer a stroke goes untreated, the greater the potential for brain damage and disability.

If you're with someone you suspect is having a stroke, watch the person carefully while waiting for emergency assistance.

Taking aspirin isn't advised during a stroke because not all strokes are caused by blood clots. Some strokes are caused by ruptured blood vessels and taking aspirin could make these bleeding strokes more severe.

Sudden Cardiac Arrest

CPR (Cardiopulmonary Resuscitation) is an emergency lifesaving procedure performed when the heart stops beating. Immediate CPR can triple chances of survival after cardiac arrest. Sudden cardiac arrest is the abrupt loss of heart function, breathing and consciousness; the condition usually results from a problem with your heart's electrical system, which disrupts your heart's pumping action and stops blood flow to your body.

Sudden cardiac arrest isn't the same as a heart attack. A heart attack is when blood flow to a part of the heart is blocked; whereas cardiac arrest is when the heart's electrical system malfunctions. However, a heart attack can sometimes trigger an electrical disturbance that leads to sudden cardiac arrest.

If not treated immediately, sudden cardiac arrest can lead to death. Survival is possible with fast, appropriate medical care. Cardiopulmonary resuscitation (CPR), using a defibrillator — or even just giving compressions to the chest — can improve the chances of survival until emergency workers arrive.

- Sudden cardiac arrest is a leading cause of death in the United States, claiming more than 350,000 lives each year.
- Approximately 90% of those who experience sudden cardiac arrest do not survive.
- Cardiac arrest kills more than 1,000 people a day, or one person every 90 seconds.
- Cardiovascular disease is the leading cause of death in the U.S. and most

deaths from it are attributable to cardiac arrest, where the heart abruptly and unexpectedly ceases to beat so that no blood can be pumped to the rest of the body.

· The most common cause of cardiac arrest is a heart rhythm disorder (arrhythmia) called ventricular fibrillation (VF). VF is an "electrical problem" in the heart. Without immediate emergency help, death follows within minutes of an episode of ventricular fibrillation.

· Cardiac arrest most often occurs in patients with heart disease, especially those who have congestive heart failure and have had a heart attack.

· It is estimated that 90 percent of victims who experience cardiac arrest die before they reach a hospital or some other source of emergency help.

· Cardiac arrest is not a random event. Although it may occur in outwardly healthy people, most victims do have heart disease or other health problems, often without being aware of it.

Emergency Treatment of Cardiac Arrest

· Ensure scene safety.
· Check for response.
· Shout for help. Tell someone nearby to call 911 or your emergency response number.
· Check for no breathing or only gasping. If the person isn't breathing or is only gasping, begin CPR.
· Use an AED, if necessary and available.

CPR (Cardiopulmonary Resuscitation)

When should you start CPR?

They are not breathing:

- If the person is not breathing, it's time to perform CPR to circulate oxygenated blood through the body. Without blood flow and oxygen the heart stops beating and the brain starts dying. *The average person can only go without oxygen between 4-6 minutes before irreversible damage is done to the brain.* If you start CPR within that time frame after cardiac arrest, there is hope that a person will survive without brain damage.

They take occasional gasping breaths:

- When someone goes into cardiac arrest they may continue to breathe for a while. If they occasionally gasp for breath, CPR compressions should be started right away.

The heart has stopped beating:

- If you cannot feel a pulse, begin performing CPR. If the heart isn't pumping oxygen is not getting to the rest of the body. Chest compressions keep blood flowing to the heart and brain until emergency responders can take over and try other methods of resuscitation.

If you are afraid to do CPR, know that it's always better to try than to do nothing. The difference between doing something and doing nothing could be someone's life.

Hands-Only CPR

- Check to make sure the scene is safe.
- Tap the person on the shoulder to see if they are responsive. Look for signs of rhythmic, normal breathing.
- If the person is non-responsive tap or shake his or her shoulder and ask loudly, "Are you OK?"
- If the person doesn't respond and is not breathing, it's time to perform CPR.
- Begin CPR. NOTE: As soon as an AED is available, deliver one shock if instructed by the device, then begin CPR.
- Put the person on his or her back on a firm surface.
- Kneel next to the person's chest.
- Place the lower palm (heel) of your hand over the center of the person's chest, between the nipples.
- Place your other hand on top of the first hand. Keep your elbows straight and position your shoulders directly above your hands.
- Push straight down (compress) on the chest at least 2 inches (5 centimeters), but no more than 2.4 inches (6 centimeters). Use your body weight (not just your arms) when doing compressions.
- Push hard at a rate of 100 to 120 compressions per minute. The American Heart Association (AHA) suggests performing compressions to the beat of the Bee Gees' song "Stayin' Alive." Allow the chest to spring back (recoil) after each push.
- Continue chest compressions until there are signs of movement or until

emergency medical personnel take over.

If you are alone and didn't see the collapse, start chest compressions for about two minutes; then quickly call 911 or your local emergency number and get the AED if one is available.

If you are alone and you did see the person collapse, call 911 number first; then get the AED, if available, and start CPR.

If another person is with you, have that person call for help and get the AED while you start CPR.

CPR with rescue breaths

- Kneel next to the person.
- Use your fingers to locate the end of the person's breastbone, where the ribs come together.
- Place two fingers at the tip of the breastbone.
- Place the heel of the other hand right above your fingers (on the side closest to the person's face).
- Use both hands to give chest compressions. Stack your other hand on top of the one that you just put in position. Lace the fingers of both hands together and raise your fingers so they do not touch the chest.
- After every 30 chest compressions, give 2 rescue breaths.
- Tilt the person's head gently and lift the chin up with 2 fingers. Pinch the person's nose. Seal your mouth over their mouth and blow steadily and firmly into their mouth for about 1 second. Give 2 rescue breaths. Check that their chest rises. If no chest rise, re-tilt the head to try to establish an open airway.
- Continue with cycles of 30 chest compressions and 2 rescue breaths until they begin to recover or emergency help arrives.

Head Tilt–Chin Lift Maneuver

To open a patient's airway using the head tilt–chin lift maneuver, place one hand on the patient's forehead and place the fingers of your other hand under the bony part of the lower jaw near the chin. Push down on the forehead and lift up and forward on the chin. Be certain you are not merely pushing the mouth closed when you use this maneuver.

- Place the patient on his or her back and kneel beside the patient.
- Place one hand on the patient's forehead and apply firm pressure.
- Backward with your palm, move the patient's head back as far as possible.
- Place the tips of the fingers of your other hand under the bony part of the lower jaw near the chin.
- Lift the chin forward to help tilt back the head.

Jaw-Thrust Maneuver

The jaw-thrust maneuver is another way to open a patient's airway. If a patient has a suspected neck injury, tilting the head may cause permanent paralysis. If you suspect a neck injury, first try to open the airway using the jaw-thrust maneuver. Open the airway by placing your fingers under the angles of the jaw and pushing upward. At the same time, use your thumbs to open the mouth slightly. The jaw-thrust maneuver should open the airway without extending the neck.

- Carefully place the patient on his or her back and kneel at the top of the patient's head.
- Place your fingers behind the angles of the patient's lower jaw and move the jaw forward with firm pressure.
- Tilt the head backward to a neutral or slight sniffing position. Do not extend the cervical spine in a patient who has sustained an injury to the head or neck.
- Use your thumbs to pull down the patient's lower jaw, opening the mouth

enough to allow breathing through the mouth and nose.

- If you are unable to open the patient's airway using the jaw-thrust maneuver, try the head tilt–chin lift maneuver as a secondary attempt to open the patient's airway.

Check for Fluids, Foreign Bodies, or Dentures

After you have opened the patient's airway by using either the head tilt–chin lift or the jaw-thrust maneuver, look in the patient's mouth to see if anything is blocking the patient's airway. Potential blocks include secretions, such as vomit, mucus or blood; foreign objects, such as candy, food or dirt; or dentures/false teeth that may have become dislodged and are blocking the patient's airway. If you find anything in the patient's mouth, remove it.

Finger Sweeps

Finger sweeps can be done quickly and require no special equipment except a set of medical gloves.

- Turn the patient onto his or her side.
- Insert your gloved fingers into the patient's mouth.
- Curve your fingers into a C-shape and sweep them from one side of the back of the mouth to the other side. Scoop out as much of the foreign material as possible. A gauze pad wrapped around your gloved fingers may help remove the obstructing materials.
- Repeat the finger sweeps until you have removed all the foreign material in the patient's mouth.

Mouth-to-Mouth Rescue Breathing

Mouth-to-mouth rescue breathing is an effective way of providing artificial ventilation for patients who are not breathing and requires no equipment except you. However, because there is a somewhat higher risk of contracting a disease when using this method, use a mask or barrier breathing device if available.

- Open the airway with the head tilt–chin lift maneuver. Press on the forehead to maintain the backward tilt of the head.
- Pinch the patient's nostrils together with your thumb and forefinger.
- Keep the patient's mouth open with the thumb of whichever hand you are using to lift the patient's chin.
- Take a deep breath and then make a tight seal by placing your mouth over the patient's mouth.
- Breathe slowly into the patient's mouth for 1 second. Breathe until the patient's chest rises.
- Remove your mouth and allow the patient to exhale passively.
- Check to see that the patient's chest falls after each exhalation.

Face Shield

A face shield is made of a tough plastic sheet that is water-tight and has a built-in masterpiece that works as a one-way valve. The barrier is simply placed on top of the victim's face during CPR, covering both mouth and nose. One end of the mouthpiece is inserted in the victim's mouth while the responder blows air through the other end. Ensure that the flat plastic stays between responder and victim to avoid transmission.

Face Mask

A face mask is a moulded plastic that fits over the person's face and has a longer one-way valve. When used correctly, it can create a tight seal during resuscitation using an inflated bladder that sits on the victim's face. The strap that goes over the rescuer's face will ensure the mask stays in place. Upon blowing air into the one-way valve, it will fill the sealed mask with oxygen that goes directly to the patient.

Bag Valve Mask

There is a little more to ventilating a patient than just squeezing the bag-valve mask. If you are squeezing the bag, but the airway is not open, you are not doing much good. Before you place the mask over the patient's nose and mouth, be sure to open the airway. If there is not a suspected neck or spine injury, use the head tilt-chin lift method. In the case of a spine injury, use the jaw thrust method, which involves moving the lower jaw forward without tilting the head back. After the airway is open, hold the mask over the nose and mouth using you thumb and index finger, which should form a "**C**" shape. Use your other fingers to hold the patient's head in the proper position. Each breath should take about 1 second.

CPR on children

You should carry out CPR with rescue breaths on a child. It's more likely children will have a problem with their airways and breathing than a problem with their heart.

Children over 1 year

- Open the child's airway by placing 1 hand on their forehead and gently tilting their head back and lifting the chin. Remove any visible obstructions from their mouth and nose.
- Pinch the child's nose and seal your mouth over their mouth, blow steadily and firmly into their mouth, checking that their chest rises. Give 5 initial rescue breaths.
- Place the heel of 1 hand on the center of the child's chest and push down by 5cm (about 2 inches), which is approximately one-third of the chest diameter. The quality (depth) of chest compressions is very important. Use 2 hands if you can't achieve a depth of 5cm using 1 hand.
- After every 30 chest compressions at a rate of 100 to 120 a minute, give 2

breaths.

- Continue with cycles of 30 chest compressions and 2 rescue breaths until the child begins to recover or emergency help arrives.

Infants under 1 year

- Open the infant's airway by placing 1 hand on their forehead and gently tilting the head back and lifting their chin. Remove any visible obstructions from their mouth and nose.
- Place both thumbs (side-by-side) on the center of the baby's chest, just below the nipple line. Use the other fingers to encircle the baby's chest toward the back, providing support. Using both thumbs at the same time, push hard down and fast about 1 ½ inches at a rate of 100 to 120 per minute. Allow the chest to return to its normal position after each compression
- *Alternatively*, you can use th+e two-finger technique. Place 2 fingers in the middle of the infant's chest and push down by 4cm (about 1.5 inches), which is approximately one-third of the chest diameter. Find the right position for chest compressions by drawing an imaginary line between the nipples to find the middle of the breastbone.
- After 30 chest compressions at a rate of 100 to 120 a minute, give 2 rescue breaths. Place your mouth over the infant's mouth and nose and blow steadily and firmly into their mouth, checking that their chest rises.
- Continue with cycles of 30 chest compressions and 2 rescue breaths until the infant begins to recover or emergency help arrives.

Two-person CPR

Two-person CPR can be extremely advantageous. When 2 people offer resuscitation, one person can obtain the AED and call for emergency services while the other administers high-quality chest compressions and rescue breaths.

Additionally, one rescuer can offer chest compressions while the other provides rescue breaths. Furthermore, the two rescuers can switch between offering chest compressions to avoid fatigue and ensure that compressions are always high-quality.

If you're offering two-person CPR, make sure that you're counting off your chest compressions out loud and yelling "Switch!" when you need the other person to begin offering chest compressions in your place (ideally after 5 cycles). Also, make sure you're vocalizing if you're getting too tired to continue delivering high-quality chest compressions and always minimize interruptions in chest compressions by switching roles as quickly as possible.

When should you stop giving CPR

Sometimes the person who needed your help may not anymore. You were right to perform CPR, but you also need to know when to stop before hurting someone. Stop if and when:

- The person becomes responsive and their condition is stable again. If the person you are helping regains consciousness or begins to breathe normally on their own, stop giving CPR. It means that your efforts were a success!
- The area becomes unsafe or unstable. What may have started out as a safe place to perform CPR may become dangerous. If the location becomes dangerous, you need to take care of yourself. You did everything you could, but putting yourself in harm's way isn't going to help anyone.
- Emergency personnel arrives. Once the professionals arrive, continue what you are doing and follow any directions that they give. They know what they are doing and have the equipment that you don't; let them do their job.
- An AED becomes available. It dramatically increases survivability when used with CPR. If indicated, an AED should be used throughout the

resuscitation.

- If you cannot physically continue to perform compression it's appropriate to stop CPR. Stopping CPR due to fatigue is protected under the Good Samaritan law.

Knowing when and when not to perform CPR drastically increases the chances that you save someone's life. If done properly, CPR can bring a person back from the dead and help them go on to live normal lives.

Circumstances that may make CPR inappropriate

The rule is, when in doubt, always begin CPR.

Obvious Death

When you witness cardiac arrest, starting CPR immediately gives the victim the highest chance of survival. However, sometimes cardiac arrest is not witnessed and the victim is found unresponsive after an unknown amount of hours. It's also possible the deceased may have non-viable injuries, such as catastrophic brain trauma. When discovering an unresponsive victim, one must assess the person to see if starting CPR is necessary. Here are the signs to look for:

Cold To the Touch

If you touch a person and they are very cold to the touch, this is usually an indication that they are beyond the point of being revived by CPR. However, surroundings should be taken into account. If a person is outside in cold weather or a drowning victim, they may be examples of where feeling the skin could give false indications.

In contrast, bodies found in bed with several layers of blankets over them.

While they may have been dead for hours, their skin will generally feel very warm. These things should be taken into account when assessing when to start CPR.

Rigor Mortis

Latin: *rigor* "stiffness", *mortis* "of death". The third stage of death, is one of the recognizable signs of death, caused by chemical changes in the muscles post mortem, which cause the limbs of the corpse to stiffen. In humans, rigor mortis can occur as soon as 4 hours post mortem.

Livor Mortis (Lividity)

"Livor" refers to the bluish color you'll find on someone who has been deceased for several hours. It is caused by blood settling and eventually permeating the skin. It resembles bruising, but will cover large portions of the body.

Lividity always occurs at a person's center of gravity. For example, if someone is lying face down, they will generally have lividity on their face and front torso. This sign can commonly be hidden either by clothes or is only seen when the person is rolled over. Regardless, if lividity is recognized, it is a definitive sign of death.

Injuries Not Compatible With Life

These kind of injuries are significant and will overrule even the best attempts of CPR. Examples of this would be decapitation, amputations of the torso, etc. Some EMS services have protocols which discourage paramedics from starting CPR on any major traumatic arrests. A traumatic arrest is when someone has a trauma such as an amputation that causes them to bleed excessively and to the point that their heart goes into cardiac arrest. Performing CPR is counter-intuitive in this circumstance because there is no blood to circulate with compressions and no red blood cells to carry oxygen from rescue breaths.

Ice cold water drowning victims can be brought back to life up to two hours after they drown if the right steps are taken; even if the heart has stopped beating and the victims' brain isn't getting the oxygen it needs to stay alive. Extremely cold water triggers something called the "mammalian diving response." Research shows the key is to start CPR immediately. Once victims reach the hospital, doctors can slowly warm and restore blood flow, often bringing the dead back to life.

A person struck by lightning may appear dead, with no pulse or breath. Often the person can be revived with cardio-pulmonary resuscitation (CPR). There is no danger to anyone helping a person who has been struck by lightning – no electric charge remains. CPR should be attempted immediately.

Complications of CPR

Aspiration & Vomiting

The most frequent occurrence during CPR is vomiting. It can present a danger to the cardiac arrest victim. Since the cardiac arrest victim is unconscious, he cannot clear the vomit from his mouth. If not cleared, the victim is likely to aspirate (inhale) it into his lungs, blocking the airway and leading to possible infection. When they vomit, turn them on their side IMMEDIATELY and remove the barrier device. When they are finished, turn them back down and continue. Just because they vomit does not mean they have been revived, it simply means your cycle was interrupted and when they are finished you must continue.

Broken Ribs Bone

Ribs can fracture as the result of CPR chest compressions. So, what do you do if you hear or feel a bone cracking underneath your hands during CPR compressions? You keep going. A significant portion of the people who receive cardiopulmonary resuscitation end up with broken ribs or other bones. If you need to perform CPR on a patient, don't be afraid of breaking their ribs.

Abdominal Distension

Another common side effect is Abdominal Distension. The abdomen of the patient becomes distended (bloated) and full of air leading to pressure on the lungs (making ventilation more difficult) and an increased chance of vomiting.

If their heart is stopped that means they are dead. Can you hurt someone worse than dead.

AED (Automated External Defibrillators)

An **automated external defibrillator** (**AED**) is a portable electronic device that automatically diagnoses the life-threatening cardiac arrhythmias of ventricular fibrillation (VF) and pulseless ventricular tachycardia, and is able to treat them through defibrillation, the application of electricity which stops the arrhythmia, allowing the heart to re-establish an effective rhythm. With simple audio and visual commands, AEDs are designed to be simple to use for the layperson, who ideally should have received AED training.

When turned on or opened, the AED will instruct the user to connect the electrodes (pads) to the patient. Once the pads are attached, everyone should avoid touching the patient so as to avoid false readings by the unit. The pads allow the AED to examine the electrical output from the heart and determine if the patient is in a shockable rhythm (either ventricular fibrillation or ventricular tachycardia). If the device determines that a shock is warranted, it will use the battery to charge its internal capacitor in preparation to deliver the shock. The device system is not only safer, charging only when required, but also allows for a faster delivery of the electric current.

- **Turn on the AED** and follow audio instructions.
- **Remove all clothing** surrounding the patient's chest (including bra).
- **Apply the <u>electrode pads</u> (included)** to the person's bare skin. Make sure the person's chest is dry.
- **Allow the AED to analyze the person's heart rhythm.** Make sure no one, including you, is touching the victim. Touching the victim can interrupt

the AED's analysis.

- **Deliver a shock (if needed).**   If the AED determines that the patient is in cardiac arrest and that a shock is needed, the way it delivers the shock depends on whether the AED is a semi-automatic model or a fully-automatic model.

Fully-automatic AED: if a shock is required it will charge and tell you to stand clear from the patient. Then it will count down and automatically deliver the shock without requiring you to press a button.

Semi-automatic AED: if a shock is required, it will charge and, once ready to deliver a shock, prompt you to push a button. The button is usually flashing and easy to locate in the middle of an emergency, but make sure you don't accidentally press the power button.

Make sure no one touches the person as the AED delivers a defibrillation shock.

- **Perform CPR and re-analyze.** AEDs are programmed with the American Heart Association's (AHA) guidelines. The current AHA's protocols call for two minutes of CPR in between AED heart rhythm analysis periods. Follow the AED instructions about when to resume CPR and when to deliver additional shocks.
- **Continue listening to the AED until EMS arrives and takes over the rescue.**

How to Use an AED on a Child

To use an AED on a child, you need to determine whether or not the AED requires a separate set of child electrode pads or if the AED has a built-in attenuator. For the most part, pediatric electrode pads work the same way as standard adult electrode pads; by enabling the AED to analyze a patient's heart and, if needed, helping deliver a lifesaving shock generated by the defibrillator to the child's body.

When the patient is a child, the energy level of the shock is attenuated ("reduced") from the standard adult energy setting. In most cases, the energy is decreased from 150 joules used for adults to 50 joules. Depending on an AED's make and model, the attenuation might be pre-set into a separate set of pediatric electrode pads, built for the sole and exclusive use of pediatric patients, or it might be built into the AED and activated using a button, "key," or another switching mechanism. If your AED requires a separate set of electrodes, you will need to install the child pads during the emergency, power on the AED, and listen to the voice prompts just like you would for an adult patient. If your AED allows you to use the same pads for adult and pediatric patients, you only need to change the device to child or pediatric mode on your AED.

If infant or pediatric settings and pads are not available, rescuers may use adult pads on infants and young children.

- **Turn on the AED** and follow the audio instructions.
- **Remove all clothing** surrounding the patient's chest and ensure the skin is dry.
- **Press the child button** or insert the child key into the AED (if the unit has one)
- **Attach the pediatric pads**, if available.

Usually, the proper location to attach AED pads on a child is anterior-posterior (or "front-and-back") placement – which is when one electrode pad is placed in the center of the child's chest and the other pad is placed in the center of their back.

Be sure to check your AED's owner's manual for specific electrode pad placement instructions. If you can't find it there, most AEDs have an image printed directly on the electrode pads that signify where they should be placed on the patient's body.

- **Allow the AED to analyze** the child's heart rhythm.
- **Deliver a shock (if needed).** If the AED determines that the patient is in cardiac arrest and that a shock is needed. Make sure no one touches the person as the AED delivers a defibrillation shock.
- **Perform CPR and re-analyze.** AEDs are programmed with the American Heart Association's guidelines. The current AHA's protocols call for two-minutes of CPR in between AED heart rhythm analysis periods. Follow the AED instructions.
- **Continue listening to the AED until EMS arrives and takes over the rescue.**

Just as with the adult process, if the AED does not find a shockable rhythm, continue with CPR until paramedics arrive.

Can You Use an AED on Someone with a Pacemaker

AED pads should not come in contact with the pacemaker device. This is relatively easy since most pacemakers are implanted in an individual's chest, and the AED pads go on the upper right and lower left rib cage. As long as you are using the AED properly, there shouldn't be any cause for concern.

Can You Use an AED in Water

No! Since AEDs deliver an electrical shock, you must take specific care when treating cardiac arrest victims who have been submerged in water. When using a defibrillator on someone who has been submerged in water, it's crucial to get the person on dry land first. You cannot apply the AED pads, which deliver the necessary electrical shock to the victim's chest, until the shirt has been removed and the skin dried thoroughly. Once the person's skin is dry, power on the AED and follow its instructions the same way you would during a normal response.

For successful defibrillation the electricity needs to flow from one electrode pad to the other, going through the chest. If the pads aren't stuck on properly the charge of electricity will flow across the chest instead of through it. Not only will this be ineffective treatment it could also cause sparks and fire to start.

Defibrillators cannot be used over clothing or on moist skin either. The patient's chest must be dried before attempting defibrillation and all clothes on the chest must be taken off, even bras. If their hair is too excessive, it can actually prevent the pads from sticking to their skin. Defibrillators come with ready kits that include a razor, to shave body hair, and tough cut scissors, to take the patients' clothes off when the defibrillator needs to be administered.

It is perfectly safe to use a defibrillator on a metal surface – providing the pads have been applied correctly and the chest is dry,

Choking / Obstructed Airway

Relieving a foreign body airway obstruction requires no special equipment. The following sections describe the steps that you need to learn to relieve foreign body airway obstructions in adults, children, and infants. Performing these steps can make the difference between life and death for these patients.

Airway Obstruction in an Adult

- Ask, "Are you choking? Can you speak? Can I help you?" If there is no verbal response, assume the airway obstructed.
- Stand behind the patient and position the thumb side of your fist just above the patient's navel.
- Press into the patient's abdomen with a quick, upward thrust. Repeat the abdominal thrusts until either the foreign body is expelled or the patient becomes unresponsive.
- If the patient is obese or is in the late stages of pregnancy, use chest thrusts instead of abdominal thrusts. Chest thrusts are done by standing behind the patient and placing your arms under the patient's armpits to encircle the patient's chest. Press with quick, backward thrusts.
- If the patient becomes unresponsive, continue with the following steps.
- **Call 911.**
- Begin CPR.
- Open the airway and look in the mouth. Remove any visible foreign body (do not attempt to remove anything unless you can see it).
- Attempt rescue breathing. If you are unable to ventilate, reposition the

patient's head and reattempt. If both breaths do not produce visible chest rise, continue chest compressions.
- Continue CPR until EMS personnel arrive.

Studies have shown that performing chest compressions on an unresponsive patient increases the pressure in the chest similar to performing abdominal thrusts and may relieve an airway obstruction. Therefore, performing CPR on a patient who has become unresponsive has the same effect as performing the Heimlich maneuver on a conscious patient.

Airway Obstruction in a Child

The steps for relieving an airway obstruction in a conscious child (age 1 year to the onset of puberty) are the same as for an adult patient. The anatomic differences between adults, children and infants require that you make some adjustments in your technique. When opening the airway of a child or infant, tilt the head back just past the neutral position. Tilting the head too far back (hyperextending the neck) can actually obstruct the airway of a child or infant.

Airway Obstruction in an Infant

The process for relieving an airway obstruction in an infant (younger than 1 year) must take into consideration that an infant is extremely fragile. An infant's airway structures are very small, and they are more easily injured than those of an adult. If you suspect an airway obstruction, assess the infant to determine whether there is any air exchange. If the infant has an audible cry, the airway is not completely obstructed. Ask the person who was with the infant what was happening when the episode began. This person may have seen the infant put a foreign body into his or her mouth. Suspect a severe airway obstruction if you observe no movement of air from the infant's mouth and nose, a sudden onset of severe breathing difficulty, a silent cough, or a silent cry. To relieve an airway obstruction in an infant, use a combination of back slaps and chest thrusts. You must have a good grasp of the infant to alternate the back slaps and the chest thrusts. Review the following sequence until you can carry it out automatically. To assist a conscious infant with a severe airway obstruction, you must:

- Assess the infant's airway and breathing status. Determine that there is no air exchange.
- Place the infant in a face down position over one arm so you can deliver five back slaps. Support the infant's head and neck with one hand and place the infant face down with the head lower than the trunk.
- Rest the infant on your forearm and support your forearm on your thigh. Use the heel of your hand and deliver up to five back slaps forcefully between the infant's shoulder blades.
- Support the head and turn the infant face up by sandwiching the infant between your hands and arms. Rest the infant on his or her back with the head lower than the trunk.
- Deliver five chest thrusts in the middle of the sternum. Use two fingers to deliver the chest thrusts in a firm manner.
- Repeat the series of back slaps and chest thrusts until the foreign object is expelled or until the infant becomes unresponsive.

If the infant becomes unresponsive, continue with the following steps

- Call 911.
- Begin CPR. Perform chest compressions. Open the airway and look in the mouth. Remove the foreign body only if you can see it. Attempt to ventilate with rescue breaths. If you are unable to ventilate, reposition the patient's head and reattempt ventilation. If both breaths do not produce visible chest rise, continue chest compressions.
- Continue CPR until EMS personnel arrive.

Don't die of politeness – if you find yourself choking, don't get embarrassed, GET ATTENTION! A lot of choking victims die in restaurant bathrooms

because they tried to clear their airways by themselves in private. Don't let this be you - make a fuss if you need help!

Opioid Overdose

Opioid use can lead to death due to the effects of opioids on the part of the brain which regulates breathing. An opioid overdose can be identified by a combination of three signs and symptoms

- Pinpoint pupils
- Unconsciousness
- Difficulties with breathing

There are a number of risk factors for opioid overdose

- Having an opioid use disorder.
- Taking opioids by injection.
- Resumption of opioid use after an extended period of abstinence (e.g. following detoxification, release from incarceration, cessation of treatment).
- Using prescription opioids without medical supervision.
- High prescribed dosage of opioids (more than 100 mg of morphine or equivalent daily).
- Using opioids in combination with alcohol and/or other substances or medicines that suppress respiratory function such as benzodiazepines, barbiturates, anesthetics or some pain medications.
- Having concurrent medical conditions such as HIV, liver or lung diseases or mental health conditions.

Emergency responses to opioid overdose

Death following opioid overdose is preventable if the person receives basic life support and the timely administration of the drug naloxone. Naloxone is a medicine that rapidly reverses an opioid overdose. It is an opioid antagonist; this means that it attaches to opioid receptors and reverses and blocks the effects of other opioids. Naloxone can quickly restore normal breathing to a person if their breathing has slowed or stopped because of an opioid overdose. But, naloxone has no effect on someone who does not have opioids in their system, and it is not a treatment for opioid use disorder. Examples of opioids include heroin, fentanyl, oxycodone (OxyContin®), hydrocodone (Vicodin®), codeine and morphine. Naloxone has virtually no effect in people who have not taken opioids. Several countries have introduced naloxone as over-the-counter medication and have also started proactive dissemination in communities.

How is naloxone given?

Naloxone should be given to any person who shows signs of an opioid overdose or when an overdose is suspected. Naloxone can be given as a nasal spray or it can be injected into the muscle or into the veins.

Naloxone works to reverse opioid overdose in the body for only 30 to 90 minutes. But many opioids remain in the body longer than that. Because of this, it is possible for a person to still experience the effects of an overdose after a dose of naloxone wears off. Also, some opioids are stronger and might require multiple doses of naloxone. Therefore, one of the most important steps to take is to call 911 so the individual can receive immediate medical attention.

Where can I get naloxone?

Many pharmacies carry naloxone. In some states, you can get naloxone from a pharmacist even if your doctor did not write you a prescription for it. It is also possible to get naloxone from community-based distribution programs, local public health groups, or local health departments, free of charge.

Recovery Position

If the patient is breathing but not fully conscious, and if no other injuries are present, you can place them in the recovery position while you wait for emergency personnel.

- Kneel beside them. Make sure they are face up and straighten their arms and legs.
- Take the arm closest to you and fold it over their chest.
- Take the arm farthest from you and extend it away from the body.
- Bend the leg closest to you at the knee.
- Support the patient's head and neck with one hand. Hold the bent knee, and roll the person away from you.
- Tilt the patient's head back to keep the airway clear and open.

Who Should Not Be Put in the Recovery Position

The recovery position is widely used in first aid situations, but there are some situations when it is not appropriate. In some cases, moving a patient on their side or moving them at all could make their injury worse.

Do not use the recovery position if the patient has a head, neck or spinal cord injury.

For children under age 1, place the baby face down across your forearm. Make sure to support the baby's head with your hand.

The goal of using the recovery position is to allow anything that is regurgitated to drain out of the mouth. The top of the esophagus (food pipe) is right next to the top of the trachea (windpipe). If matter comes up from the esophagus, it could easily find its way into the lungs. This could cause what is known as aspiration pneumonia, which is an infection of the lungs caused by foreign material.

Traumatic Bleeding

After a severe injury, a person can bleed out in under five minutes.

Uncontrolled post-traumatic bleeding is the leading cause of potentially preventable death among trauma patients. There are three main types of bleeding: arterial, venous and capillary bleeding. Arterial bleeding occurs in the arteries, which transport blood from the heart to the body. Venous bleeding happens in the veins, which carry blood back to the heart. Capillary bleeding takes place in the capillaries, which are tiny blood vessels that connect the arteries to the veins. *Bleeding from the arteries and veins can be severe; when this occurs, it is important for a person to receive immediate medical attention.*

Treat Non-Serious Bleeding

First, <u>apply pressure</u>! Remember, pressure stops bleeding.

How Long?

- There is no definite amount of time; just apply continuous pressure until bleeding stops.

How Much?

- Use your hands to apply firm steady pressure until bleeding stops. You should hold pressure for at least 5 minutes before looking at the wound.
- If bleeding does not stop, call 911 and continuing applying pressure until medical help arrives.
- If you can, try to ensure the injured person is on a firm surface, that way, when you apply force to the bleeding, you are pressing into something.

If you have gauze available, use it. If not, use whatever you have available, such as a shirt, newspapers, or your hand.

Uncontrolled Traumatic Bleeding

Using direct pressure and tourniquets on extremity bleeding is relatively straightforward. The bleeding in these locations is often deeper and maintaining adequate external pressure can be difficult or impossible.

Wound Packing

Wounds of the chest, abdomen or pelvis shouldn't be packed because bleeding from these wounds is generally from a very deep source that can't be reached from the outside. These patients must be rapidly transported to a surgeon for operative bleeding control.

- **Stop the bleeding.** Immediately apply direct pressure to the wound using gauze, clean cloth, or whatever you have available such as a shirt, newspapers, your hand, elbow, knee - whatever it takes to slow or stop the hemorrhage - until you have time to get out your wound packing supplies.
- Place your gloved fingers - with or without a dressing - into the wound to apply initial pressure to the target area (with your target being the vein, artery or both) and compress the source of bleeding. Keep in mind that the body's anatomy presents with major vessels running close to bones;

so, whenever possible, utilize a bone to assist with vessel (i.e., bleeding) control. This will also give you an idea of which direction the wound travels and you can insert the gauze accordingly.

· **Pack the wound with gauze – tightly!** Your goal is to completely and tightly pack the wound cavity to stop hemorrhage. Begin packing the gauze into the wound with your finger, while simultaneously maintaining pressure on the wound.

· It's critical that the gauze be packed as deeply into the wound as possible to put the gauze into direct contact with the bleeding vessel. By doing so, you're simultaneously putting direct pressure onto the bleeding vessel and allowing the hemostatic agent to do work its magic.

· **Keep packing!** The key to successful wound packing is that the wound be very tightly packed, applying as much pressure as possible to the bleeding vessel. This pressure against the vessel is the most important component of hemorrhage control. This explains why plain gauze (without an impregnated hemostatic agent), when tightly packed, is also quite effective.

· **When no more gauze can be packed inside the wound, apply very firm pressure to the packed wound for 3 minutes.** This step pushes the packing firmly against the bleeding vessel and aids in clotting.

· **Secure a snug pressure dressing.** After applying pressure for 3 minutes, place a snug pressure dressing over the wound. You may consider splinting or immobilizing the area, if possible, because movement during transport can dislodge the packing and allow hemorrhage to restart.

The biggest mistake in wound packing is being timid. Don't be shy – be bold! Pack that wound tightly! And, remember to also perform a complete assessment of your patient so as not overlook other life-threatening injuries.

Keep in mind that you won't harm the patient by deeply packing a wound, you'll help them.

Applying a Tourniquet

A tourniquet is a device that is placed around a bleeding arm or leg. Tourniquets work by squeezing large blood vessels, which helps stop blood loss. A commercially made CAT tourniquet is preferred as these are quick and easy to use. If you don't have a commercially manufactured tourniquet, you can make one using a strip of soft material 2–4 inches wide and a sturdy stick. Tie the stick into the material and twist to tighten the tourniquet.

How do I use a Tourniquet?

- Send someone to **call 911** and have someone apply pressure to the wound using a clean gauze or cloth.
- Place the tourniquet around the wounded limb about 2 inches above the wound. Avoid placing it over a joint.
- Secure the tourniquet tightly in place.
- Twist the rod (windlass) to tighten the tourniquet until bright red bleeding stops flowing from the wound, and secure the rod in place using the clip or holder.
- Note the time you applied the tourniquet and give this information to EMS personnel when they arrive.
- **Do not remove the tourniquet**.

The experience gained over the past 15 years of combat has clearly demonstrated that recommended, commercially available tourniquets can, in fact, be used safely. Data from the U.S. military have shown that survival for trauma victims who have a tourniquet applied *before* they bleed into shock is 9 times greater than for victims who receive a tourniquet *after* they go into shock.

Shock

The sooner a shock is recognized, the better the victim's outcome will be. Although signs of shock can range greatly, some common signs are:

- A fast pulse
- Pale, cool, clammy/damp skin
- Sweating
- Flushed face
- Anxiety
- Ashen or blue skin on lips and nail beds
- Weakness and dizziness
- Nausea and possibly vomiting
- Shallow breathing
- Weak, very rapid, "thready" pulse
- Confusion or disorientation

Advanced phases:

- Lack of pulse in wrists or feet
- Restlessness and aggressiveness
- Yawning and gasping for air
- Unconsciousness

Final phase:

- Multiple organ failure
- Cardiac arrest

Treatment

The most important treatment for shock of any variety is to try to maintain the blood flow to the body's vital organs (brain, heart and lungs). To do this, lie the patient flat on the floor and raise their legs about 6–12 inches off the ground. Do not incline the victim's head, chest or pelvis, as this brings no improvement and can cause harm. Other important factors in the treatment of shock can be remembered by the simple mnemonic WART.

WART:

- Warmth
  - ABCs (Airway, Breathing, Circulation)
  - Rest and Reassurance
  - Treatment of underlying cause

Unconscious Patients

Should a patient become unconscious, reassess the ABCs. Should any change occur, compensate with required treatment. As airway takes priority over other treatment, you should place them in the recovery position in order to ensure a patent airway.

Anaphylactic Shock

Anaphylaxis is a life-threatening medical emergency because of rapid con-
striction of the airway, often within minutes of exposure to the allergen. It is
commonly triggered by insect stings and foods such as shellfish or peanuts.
Call for help immediately. First aid for anaphylaxis consists of obtaining
advanced medical care at once. Look to see if a device such as an epinephrine
autoinjector ("EpiPen") is available – most people who know they have
anaphylactic reactions will carry such a device with them. First aiders in
many jurisdictions are now permitted to administer epinephrine in the form
of an EpiPen if the victim is unable to do so themselves.

Recognition

- Hives or rash all over accompanied by itchiness
- Swelling or puffiness of the lymph nodes, especially around the neck and
  mouth
- Swelling of the airway and tongue
- Difficulty breathing, wheezing or gasping

Treatment

- **Call 911** (EMS) immediately
- Have the victim administer their epinephrine autoinjector if possible
- If available, administer an antihistamine to decrease swelling
- Encourage the victim to breathe slowly; calm them

- The victim should rest until EMS arrives
- Monitor ABCs and begin CPR if required
- If the victim is unable to administer their epinephrine autoinjector and it is legal to do so, administer it for them

Administering an Epinephrine Autoinjector

EpiPen ® **or EpiPen Jr** ® - These epinephrine autoinjectors contain one dose per autoinjector. They are available in two different doses based on the person's weight; one (brand name: EpiPen) contains 0.3 mg of epinephrine and is intended for older children and adults, and the other (brand name: EpiPen Jr) contains 0.15 mg of epinephrine and is intended for use in young children.

Auvi-Q - The Canadian version, Allerject ® epinephrine autoinjectors contain one dose per autoinjector. They are rectangular, about the size of a cell phone, and play a recording that explains each step in the self-injecting process. Auvi-Q ® autoinjectors come in three different doses: one intended for adults and older children; one intended for young children; and a third for use in infants and toddlers who weigh less than 33 lbs (15 kg).

Generic epinephrine — There are several generic versions of epinephrine autoinjectors available. These may be a lower-cost alternative to brand-name devices, and they contain the same medication. Talk to your health care provider or pharmacy if you are not sure which device you have, or if you want to know more about your options.

Other devices — Other devices may be available around the world, including some with doses higher than those available in the United States. A prefilled syringe that is not an autoinjector is also available (brand name: Symjepi ®).

How to Use

EpiPen ® - If you are about to use the autoinjector, pull up straight the blue safety release (EpiPen ® or EpiPen Jr ®) with one hand and hold the pen with the other hand. Do not flip the blue safety release off using the thumb or by pulling it sideways, or by bending and twisting it. Push the needle end (orange end of the autoinjector) firmly against the outer thigh until it "clicks". This signals that the injection has started. The autoinjector needs to stay in place for a minimum of 10 seconds following activation.

Auvi-Q ® - Voice instructions will guide you through each step of the epinephrine injection process. Push the needle end firmly against the outer thigh; AUVI-Q ® will beep, and the lights will blink red to indicate the injection is complete.

Do not remove the blue safety release (EpiPen ® or EpiPen Jr ®), the gray end caps (Adrenaclick ®), or the red safety guard (Auvi-Q®) on the autoinjector until you are ready to use it. Do not put your thumb, fingers or hand over the black base (Auvi-Q ®), orange (EpiPen ® or EpiPen Jr ®), or red (Adrenaclick ®) tip of the autoinjector or over the needle of the Symjepi ® prefilled syringe. *This is to avoid an accidental injection.*

Large-sized adults may need to repeat the dose. A second dose may also be needed if symptoms are not improving or getting worse after about five minutes, or if symptoms come back before reaching the emergency department.

Seizure

Knowing what NOT to do is important for keeping a person safe during and after a seizure.

Never do any of the following:

- Do not hold the person down or try to stop his or her movements.
- Do not put anything in the person's mouth; this can injure teeth or the jaw. A person having a seizure cannot swallow his or her tongue.
- Do not offer the person water or food until he or she is fully alert.

These are general steps to help someone who is having any type seizure:

- Ease the person to the floor.
- Clear the area around the person of anything hard or sharp.
- Put something soft and flat, like a folded jacket, under the head.
- Remove eyeglasses.
- Loosen ties or anything around the neck that may make it hard to breathe.
- Time the seizure.
- Stay with the person until the seizure ends and he or she is fully awake.
- Aid breathing by placing them in the recovery position once the jerking has stopped.
- Once they are alert and able to communicate, tell them what happened.

- Comfort the person and speak calmly.
- Check to see if the person is wearing a medical bracelet.
- Keep yourself and other people calm.
- Make sure the person gets home safely.
- If the person is in a wheelchair, put the brakes on and leave any seatbelt or harness on. Support them gently and cushion their head, but do not try to move them.

Seizures do not usually require emergency medical attention; however, seek medical care if one or more of these are true:

- The person has never had a seizure before.
- The person has difficulty breathing or waking after the seizure.
- The seizure lasts longer than 5 minutes.
- The person has another seizure soon after the first one.
- The person is hurt during the seizure.
- The seizure happens in water.
- The person has a health condition like diabetes, heart disease or is pregnant.

Having seizures in water is dangerous because of the risk of drowning - this is why swimmers with a seizure disorder should never go unsupervised.

Seizures in Water

- Gently support head so that it is above water.
- Guide to a shallower area where you can stand.
- Try not to restrain movements.
- If possible, take the person out of the water.
- Once the jerking has stopped place in the recovery position.
- Visit a medical facility to check for swallowed water.

Heat Stroke

Heat stroke occurs when the body's temperature rises rapidly, the sweating mechanism fails, and the body is unable to cool down. Body temperature may rise to 106 degrees or higher within 10 to 15 minutes. Heat stroke can cause death or permanent disability if emergency treatment is not provided.

Warning signs

- An extremely high body temperature (above 103 degrees, orally)
- Red, hot, and dry skin (no sweating)
- Rapid, strong pulse
- Throbbing headache
- Dizziness
- Nausea
- Confusion
- Unconsciousness

Treating heat stroke

- **Call 911**
- Get the victim out of the sun or heat. Move to an air-conditioned space.
- Only if fully conscious, offer water.
- Cool the victim rapidly using whatever methods you can. For example, immerse the victim in a tub of cool water; place the person in a cool shower; spray the victim with cool water from a garden hose; sponge the person

with cool water; or if the humidity is low, wrap the victim in a cool, wet sheet and fan vigorously. Cool down with ice.
· Monitor body temperature, and continue cooling efforts until the body temperature drops to 101–102 degrees.

Hypothermia

Hypothermia occurs when a person's body temperature is dangerously low. As a result, the brain and body cannot function properly. Left untreated, hypothermia can lead to cardiac arrest and death.

Symptoms of Hypothermia

- Shivering and chattering teeth
- Exhaustion
- Clumsiness, slow movements and reactions; prone to falling
- Sleepiness
- Weak pulse
- Fast heart rate
- Rapid breathing
- Pale skin color
- Confusion and poor judgment/loss of awareness
- Excessive urination
- Slowdown in breathing and heart rate
- Slurred speech
- Decline in mental function
- Loss of shivering
- Bluish color to skin
- Muscle stiffness
- Dilated pupils
- Abnormal heart rhythm

- Decreased blood pressure
- Weakened reflexes
- Loss of consciousness
- Low blood pressure
- Fluid in lungs
- Absence of reflexes
- Low urine output
- Heart stops beating (cardiac arrest)
- Coma that may mimic death
- Death

Treating hypothermia

- **Call 911**
- Gently move the person out of the cold. If going indoors isn't possible, protect the person from the wind, especially around the neck and head. Insulate the individual from the cold ground.
- Gently remove wet clothing. Replace wet things with warm, dry coats or blankets.
- If further warming is needed, do so gradually. For example, apply warm, dry compresses to the center of the body (neck, chest and groin). The CDC says another option is using an electric blanket, if available. If you use hot water bottles or a chemical hot pack, first wrap it in a towel before applying.
- Offer the person warm, sweet, nonalcoholic drinks.

CAUTION

- Do not rewarm the person too quickly, such as with a heating lamp or hot bath.
- Do not attempt to warm the arms and legs. Heating or massaging the limbs of someone in this condition can stress the heart and lungs.
- Do not give the person alcohol or cigarettes. Alcohol hinders the rewarm-

ing process, and tobacco products interfere with circulation that is needed for rewarming.

Begin CPR, if Necessary, While Warming Person

If the person is not breathing, start CPR immediately. Hypothermia causes respiratory rates to plunge, and a pulse might be difficult to detect, a patient isn't dead unless they are warm and dead.

Reactions to Stress

You need to understand how stress can affect you and the people for whom you provide emergency medical care. It is important to realize that a wide variety of stressful events may trigger a grief reaction. These events include a major incident, a serious illness, drug or alcohol addiction, incarceration, the end of a relationship or divorce, loss of a job or income, or a major rejection. Dying is one of the most stressful events people experience. Anyone involved with a person suffering a significant loss will go through some sort of grieving process. This includes a patient, his or her family, and caregivers, including emergency first responders.

Some people will experience grief in a variety of ways. Some people will exhibit no outward signs of grief. Other people will experience only some of the stages. People do not experience these stages of grief in any order and they can occur at any time during the grieving process.

Denial ("Not me!") - The first stage in the grieving process is denial. A person experiencing denial cannot believe what is happening. This stage may serve as a protection for the person experiencing the situation, and it may also serve as a protection for you as the caregiver. Realize that this reaction is normal.

Anger ("Why me?") - The second stage of the grieving process is anger. Understanding that anger is a normal reaction to stress can help you deal with anger that is directed toward you by a patient or the patient's family.

Do not become defensive; this anger is likely a result of the situation and
not a result of your patient care. This realization can enable you to tolerate
the situation without letting the patient's anger distract you from performing
your duties of providing care.

Bargaining ("Okay, but . . .") – The third stage of the grieving process is
bargaining. Bargaining is the act of trying to make a deal to postpone
death and dying. If you encounter a patient or family member who is in this
stage, try to respond with a truthful and helpful comment such as, "We are
doing everything we can and the paramedics will be here in just a few
minutes." Remember that bargaining may be a normal part of the grieving
process.

Depression ("Heavy-hearted") – The fourth stage of the grieving process
is depression. Depression is often characterized by sadness or despair. A
person who is unusually silent or who seems to retreat into his or her own
world may have reached this stage. This may also be the point at which a
person begins to accept the situation. It is not surprising that patients and
their families get depressed about a situation that involves death and dying
—nor is it surprising that you as a rescuer also get depressed. Our society
tends to consider death a failure of medical care rather than a natural event
that happens to everyone. A certain amount of depression is a natural
reaction to a major threat or loss. The depression can be mild or severe,
and it can be of short duration or long-lasting. If you have depression that
continues, it is important for you to contact qualified professionals who can
help you.

Acceptance – The final stage of the grieving process is acceptance.
Acceptance does not mean that you are satisfied with the situation. It
means that you understand that death and dying cannot be changed. It
may require a lot of time to work through the grieving process and arrive at
this stage. As an EMS provider, you may see acceptance in family

members who have had time to realize that their loved one's illness is terminal. However, not all people who experience grief are able to work through it and accept the loss.

By understanding these five stages, you can better understand the grief reaction experienced by patients, their families, and their friends. You can also better understand your own reaction to stressful situations.

As you go through the anger phase of the grieving process, you may want to direct your anger at the patient, the patient's family, your coworkers, or your own family. Anger is a normal reaction to unpleasant events. Sometimes it helps to talk out your anger with coworkers, family members, or a counselor – by talking through your anger, you avoid keeping it bottled up inside where it can cause unhealthy physical symptoms or emotional reactions. Directing the energy from your anger in positive ways may help you move forward. For example, at the scene of a motor vehicle crash, you may be angry that a child has been injured; but focusing your energy on providing the best medical care for the injured child may help you work through your feelings.

Stress Management

Stress management has three components:

- recognizing stress
- preventing stress
- reducing stress

An important step in managing stress in yourself and others is the ability to recognize its signs and symptoms; only then can you take steps to prevent or reduce stress.